INTRODUCTION

Kidney stones in the urinary tract are formed in several ways. Calcium can combine with chemicals, such as oxalate or phosphorous, in the urine. This can happen if these substances become so concentrated that they solidify. Kidney stones can also be caused by a buildup of uric acid. Uric acid buildup is caused by the metabolism of protein. Your urinary tract wasn't designed to expel solid matter, so it's no surprise that kidney stones are very painful to pass. Luckily, they can usually be avoided through diet.

WHAT ARE KIDNEY STONES?

Urine contains many dissolved minerals and salts. When your urine has high levels of these minerals and salts, you can form stones. Kidney stones can start small but can grow larger in size, even filling the inner hollow structures of the kidney. Some stones stay in the kidney do not

Table of Contents

cause any problems. Sometimes, the kidney stone can travel down the ureter, the tube between the kidney and the bladder. If the stone reaches the bladder, it can be passed out of the body in urine. If the stone becomes lodged in the ureter, it blocks the urine flow from that kidney and causes pain.

Kidney stones are small pieces of hard crystallized material that form in the kidney. Kidney stones are often made up of calcium, but can also contain uric acid or amino acids (proteins). Kidney stones, also called urolithiasis, are a common condition.

One or more kidney stones can form in one or both kidneys. Kidney stones begin as tiny specks and may gradually increase in size. A person with a small kidney stone may not have symptoms and may not be aware of the condition. In some cases, small stones in the urine may pass out of the kidney and move down the ureter, into the bladder, and out of the body without causing pain or serious problems.

Kidney stones form when a person's urine output decreases, and when the kidney contains large numbers of certain minerals that stick together and form stones.

Common kinds of kidney stones include:

- calcium oxalate stones
- calcium phosphate stone
- struvite stones
- uric acid stones
- cystine stones

A range of factors can cause kidney stones, including the following dietary factors:

- high oxalate intake from certain foods
- a high protein diet
- too much sodium

- dehydration or low fluid intake

High oxalate foods, such as nuts, seeds, beets, spinach, and buckwheat flour, can contribute to calcium oxalate stones, although this does not mean that people need to exclude them from the diet completely.

A high protein diet can contribute to the formation of calcium phosphate stones. A high sodium intake and dehydration can contribute to uric acid and cystine stones.

WHAT IS THE KIDNEY STONE DIET?

Drinking plenty of water is an aspect of the kidney stone diet.

People who wish to prevent kidney stones developing for the first time or reduce the risk of recurrence if they have already had stones should follow these main steps:

- drink plenty of water
- limit their intake of salt and animal protein
- restrict foods that contain high levels of oxalates
- get enough calcium

There is no single diet plan for all types of kidney stones, as they can form due to a buildup of several different minerals in the body. However, many dietitians and doctors who specialize in kidney diseases, or nephrologists, recommend the Dietary Approaches to Stop Hypertension (DASH) diet for people with kidney stones.

This diet has demonstrated the ability to reduce the risk of kidney stone formation and improve other elements of overall health, such as lower blood pressure and a reduced risk of heart disease, stroke, and cancer.

The DASH diet encourages people to consume vegetables, fruits, whole grains, and low-fat dairy. The plan also suggests limiting the intake of salt, sugar, and red meat.

However, dietary changes mainly affect people at risk of the following types of kidney stone:

- calcium oxalate stones
- calcium phosphate stones
- uric acid stones
- cystine stones

People should speak with their healthcare provider to work out which type of kidney stones they have had, if any, to support effective dietary choices. The National Kidney Foundation recommend cutting back on sodium in the diet rather than reducing calcium intake.

THE KIDNEYS AND URINARY SYSTEM

The kidneys are fist-size organs that handle the body's fluid and chemical levels. Most people have two kidneys, one on each side of the spine behind the liver, stomach, pancreas and intestines. Healthy kidneys clean waste from the blood and remove it in the urine. They control the levels of sodium, potassium and calcium in the blood.

The kidneys, ureters and bladder are part of your urinary tract. The urinary tract makes, transports, and stores urine in the body. The kidneys make urine from water and your body's waste. The urine then travels down the ureters into the bladder, where it is stored. Urine leaves your body through the urethra.

Kidney stones form in the kidney. Some stones move from the kidney into the ureter. The ureters are tubes leading from the kidneys to the bladder. If a stone leaves the kidney and gets stuck in the ureter, it is called a ureteral stone.

WHAT ARE KIDNEY STONES MADE OF?

Kidney stones come in many different types and colors. How you treat them and stop new stones from forming depends on what type of stone you have.

Calcium stones (80 percent of stones)

Calcium stones are the most common type of kidney stone. There are two types of calcium stones: calcium oxalate and calcium phosphate. Calcium oxalate is by far the most common type of calcium stone. Some people have too much calcium in their urine, raising their risk of calcium stones. Even with normal amounts of calcium in the urine, calcium stones may form for other reasons.

Uric acid stones (5-10 percent of stones)

Uric acid is a waste product that comes from chemical changes in the body. Uric acid crystals do not dissolve well in acidic urine and instead will form a uric acid stone. Having acidic urine may come from:

- Being overweight
- Chronic diarrhea
- Type 2 diabetes (high blood sugar)
- Gout
- A diet that is high in animal protein and low in fruits and vegetables

Struvite/infection stones (10 percent of stones)

Struvite stones are not a common type of stone. These stones are related to chronic urinary tract infections (UTIs). Some bacteria make the urine less acidic and more basic or alkaline. Magnesium ammonium phosphate (struvite) stones form in alkaline urine. These stones are often large, with branches, and they often grow very fast.

People who get chronic UTIs, such as those with long-term tubes in their kidneys or bladders, or people with poor bladder emptying due to neurologic disorders (paralysis, multiple sclerosis, and spina bifida) are at the highest risk for developing these stones.

Cystine stones (less than 1 percent of stones)

Cystine is an amino acid that is in certain foods; it is one of the building blocks of protein. Cystinuria (too much cystine in the urine) is a rare, inherited metabolic disorder. It is when the kidneys do not reabsorb cystine from the urine. When high amounts of cystine are in the urine, it causes stones to form. Cystine stones often start to form in childhood.

HOW DOES THE DIET WORK?

Some foods contain certain chemicals or compounds that can influence the production of kidney stones, particularly if a person regularly eats them in high amounts.

By limiting the intake of these foods, the risk of kidney stones reduces.

CAN DIET ALONE TREAT KIDNEY STONES?

For some people, dietary changes may be enough to prevent kidney stones from occurring.

In other cases, additional treatment may be necessary, including medication to break the stones up or surgery to remove the stones.

If stones become extremely painful, it is best to seek consultation with a doctor or nephrologist so they can recommend the best course of action.

DO ANY HERBAL SUPPLEMENTS HELP REDUCE THE RISK OF KIDNEY STONES?

People have used many herbs throughout time. Traditionally, people have used apple cider vinegar to prevent and treat kidney stones, and studies in the lab have shown that it can reduce the development of stones.

According to one cross-sectional study, the acetic acid in apple cider vinegar reduces pain and inflammation.

People have also used wheatgrass for centuries to improve health and because it contains certain compounds that cause increased urine output, reducing the risk that kidney stones will develop.

TYPES OF KIDNEY STONES

Knowing the type of kidney stone you have helps determine its cause and may give clues on how to reduce your risk of getting more kidney stones. If possible, try to save your kidney stone if you pass one so that you can bring it to your doctor for analysis.

Types of kidney stones include:

- **Calcium stones**. Most kidney stones are calcium stones, usually in the form of calcium oxalate. Oxalate is a substance made daily by your liver or absorbed from your diet. Certain fruits and vegetables, as well as nuts and chocolate, have high oxalate content.

- **Dietary factors**, high doses of vitamin D, intestinal bypass surgery and several metabolic disorders can increase the concentration of calcium or oxalate in urine.

- **Calcium stones** may also occur in the form of calcium phosphate. This type of stone is more common in metabolic conditions, such as renal tubular acidosis. It may also be associated with certain medications used to treat migraines or seizures, such as topiramate (Topamax, Trokendi XR, Qudexy XR).

- **Struvite stones.** Struvite stones form in response to a urinary tract infection. These stones can grow quickly and become quite large, sometimes with few symptoms or little warning.

- **Uric acid stones.** Uric acid stones can form in people who lose too much fluid because of chronic diarrhea or malabsorption, those who eat a high-protein diet, and those with diabetes or metabolic syndrome. Certain genetic factors also may increase your risk of uric acid stones.

- **Cystine stones**. These stones form in people with a hereditary disorder called cystinuria that causes the kidneys to excrete too much of a specific amino acid.

CAUSES OF KIDNEY STONES

Even if you're in good health, your diet may encourage kidney stones to grow. One top reason is you may not be drinking enough water. That means you'll make too little pee, which gives the stones more chances to form.

Other things to watch:

- Colas. These beverages are high in fructose and phosphates, which may lead to kidney stones.
- Oxalates. These are organic compounds found in a number of foods, including healthy ones such as spinach and sweet potatoes. But oxalates also bind easily to

certain minerals, including calcium, which then help form kidney stones.

- Salt (specifically, sodium). Lots of sodium, which you get mainly through salt, means more calcium in your pee. That ups your odds for kidney stones. Eating calcium-rich foods like kale and salmon is OK unless you also eat too much salt. Too little calcium in your diet may lead to kidney stones in certain people.

- Vitamin C supplements. Be careful with these. Research has found high doses of vitamin C taken regularly can double a man's chances for a kidney stone. There's no need to worry about vitamin C in food.

- Animal protein. Too many steaks, chicken, eggs, and seafood can build up calcium and uric acid in your body. That's another cause of kidney stones.

- Medications. Some prescription and over-the-counter drugs can contribute to kidney stones, including antacids, certain antibiotics, decongestants, diuretics, steroids and certain medicines for cancer, HIV, and epilepsy.
- Previous kidney stones. If you've had them once, you're likely to get them again, unless you take steps.
-

RISK FACTORS

Factors that increase your risk of developing kidney stones include:

- Family or personal history. If someone in your family has had kidney stones, you're more likely to develop stones, too. If you've already had one or more kidney stones, you're at increased risk of developing another.

- Dehydration. Not drinking enough water each day can increase your risk of kidney stones. People who live in warm, dry climates and those who sweat a lot may be at higher risk than others.

- Certain diets. Eating a diet that's high in protein, sodium (salt) and sugar may increase your risk of some types of kidney stones. This is especially true with a high-sodium diet. Too much salt in your diet increases the amount of calcium your kidneys must filter and significantly increases your risk of kidney stones.

- Obesity. High body mass index (BMI), large waist size and weight gain have been linked to an increased risk of kidney stones.

- Digestive diseases and surgery. Gastric bypass surgery, inflammatory bowel disease or chronic diarrhea can cause changes in the digestive process that affect your absorption of calcium and water, increasing the amounts of stone-forming substances in your urine.

- Other medical conditions such as renal tubular acidosis, cystinuria, hyperparathyroidism and repeated urinary tract infections also can increase your risk of kidney stones.

- Certain supplements and medications, such as vitamin C, dietary supplements, laxatives (when used excessively), calcium-based antacids, and certain medications used to treat migraines or depression, can increase your risk of kidney stones.

FOODS TO PREVENT KIDNEY STONES

Every year, more than three million people seek treatment for symptoms related to kidney stones. Many are familiar with the pain associated with kidney stones, but there are some surprising facts you might not know.

Facts About Kidney Stones

1. Calcium doesn't cause kidney stones. In moderation, eating calcium can actually help prevent stones from forming.

2. It's more common than you think. One in 10 people will develop a kidney stone in their lifetime and 85 percent will develop them again within 10 years. Men develop stones more often than women.

3. Save that stone. If you pass a stone, save it for testing. There are different types of kidney stones. By knowing what specific type of stone you had, we can tailor prevention recommendations for your individual needs.

4. One size does not fit all. Kidney stones can be as small as a grain of salt or as big as a golf ball.

Different treatments are recommended for the various sizes of stones.

5. Prevention is key. Changes in diet and medication, if indicated, are about 90 percent effective in preventing new stones from forming.

5 FOODS TO PREVENT KIDNEY STONES

Certain foods can increase your risk of developing kidney stones. Eating in moderation while maintaining a healthy diet with fruits and vegetables is encouraged. It is important to be mindful of the following foods that can lead to the formation of kidney stones in certain people: foods high in sodium, cola beverages, fast foods, processed meats, certain supplements, black tea, chocolate, spinach, soy milk, almonds, cashews, soy beans.

The good news is there are many items you can include in your regular diet to help prevent stones from occurring.

1. Water. Although a beverage and not necessarily a food, drinking water is the most important way to prevent kidney stones. We recommend two to three liters of water (at least 64 ounces or more) each day.

2. Lemon. Lemon contains citric acid that stops kidney stones from forming and helps break up stones that have already formed. For a refreshing beverage, add some fresh squeezed lemon into your water!

3. Cruciferous vegetables. Vegetables rich in potassium such as brussels sprouts, broccoli and kale decrease calcium loss and stop kidney stones from forming. These foods also have antioxidant effects that help prevent bladder, prostate and kidney cancers.

4. Whole grains. Most whole grains contribute to a healthy weight which is helpful in prevention and treatment of kidney stones.

5. Calcium. The calcium in milk and yogurt can decrease the risk of forming kidney stones.

If you have a kidney stone, we can help. The Kidney Stone Center at The Miriam Hospital is the only center of its kind in Southern New England. They use the latest technology and preventive techniques to provide comprehensive care for those who have or are recovering from kidney stones.

WHAT YOU CAN DO TO PREVENT KIDNEY STONES

If you've already had a kidney stone, your doctor may recommend medication to keep it from happening again. What kind will depend on what caused the stone.

Also, take charge of your diet:

- Drink lots of water. Stay hydrated, especially when you exercise.
- Check food labels. Read the ingredients. Avoid or cut back on foods with high amounts of ingredients like sodium chloride, monosodium glutamate (MSG), and sodium nitrate.
- Choose foods wisely. Usually it's good to get more spinach and nuts in your diet. But if you have calcium oxalate stones, which are the most common type, your doctor may tell you to avoid or limit foods high in oxalates:
- Nuts, including almonds, cashews, pistachios, and peanuts
- Soy products, including soy burgers, soy milk, and soy cheese

- Chocolate
- Oat and oat bran
- Red kidney beans, navy beans, and fava beans
- Beets, spinach, kale, and tomato

These foods are low in oxalates. Caution: Too much dairy food and animal protein can up your chances of less common types of kidney stones:

- Grapes, melons, bananas
- Cucumbers, cauliflower, cabbage, peas
- Cheese, milk, butter
- Beef, bacon, chicken, ham
- Eat citrus fruits. Lemons and limes are high in citrate, which helps prevent kidney stones.
- Get plenty of calcium. Not enough calcium in your diet can lead to kidney stones. It's better if you get it from food, like low-fat dairy products, rather than supplements.

HOME REMEDIES FOR KIDNEY STONES: WHAT WORKS?

Staying hydrated is key

Drinking plenty of fluids is a vital part of passing kidney stones and preventing new stones from forming. Not only does the liquid flush out toxins, but it also helps move stones and grit through your urinary tract.

Although water alone may be enough to do the trick, adding certain ingredients can be beneficial. Be sure to drink one 8-ounce glass of water immediately after drinking any flavored remedy. This can help move the ingredients through your system.

Talk to your doctor before getting started with any of the home remedies listed below. They can assess whether home treatment is right for you or if it could lead to additional complications.

If you're pregnant or breastfeeding, avoid using any remedies. Your doctor can determine whether a juice may cause side effects for you or your baby.

1. Water

When passing a stone, upping your water intake can help speed up the process. Strive for 12 glasses of water per day instead of the usual 8.

Once the stone passes, you should continue to drink 8 to 12 glasses of water each day. Dehydration is one of the main risk factors for kidney stones, and the last thing you want is for more to form.

Pay attention to the color of your urine. It should be a very light, pale yellow. Dark yellow urine is a sign of dehydration.

2. Lemon juice

You can add freshly squeezed lemons to your water as often as you like. Lemons contain citrate, which is a chemical that prevents calcium stones from forming. Citrate can also break up small stones, allowing them to pass more easily.

A great deal of lemons would be needed to make a huge effect, but some can help a little.

Lemon juice has numerous other health benefits. For example, it helps inhibit bacteria growth and provides vitamin C.

3. Basil juice

Basil contains acetic acid, which helps break down the kidney stones and reduce pain. It's also full of nutrients. This remedy has been used traditionally for digestive and inflammatory disorders.

There are antioxidants and anti-inflammatory agents in basil juice, and it may help maintain kidney health.

Use fresh or dried basil leaves to make a tea and drink several cups per day. You may also juice fresh basil in a juicer or add it to a smoothie.

You shouldn't use medicinal basil juice for more than 6 weeks at a time. Extended use may lead to:

- low blood sugar
- low blood pressure
- increased bleeding

There's very little research on how effective basil is for kidney stones, but it does have anti-oxidative and anti-inflammatory properties.

4. Apple cider vinegar

Apple cider vinegar contains acetic acid. Acetic acid helps dissolve kidney stones.

In addition to flushing out the kidneys, apple cider vinegar can help ease pain caused by the stones. There are numerous other health benefits of apple cider vinegar.

One lab study found that apple cider vinegar was effective in helping reduce the formation of kidney stones, though more studies are needed. But because of the numerous other health benefits, there's probably little risk.

Shop for apple cider vinegar online.

To reap these benefits, add 2 tablespoons of apple cider vinegar to 6 to 8 ounces of purified water. Drink this mixture throughout the day.

You shouldn't consume more than one 8-ounce glass of this mixture per day. You can also use it on salads straight or add it to your favorite salad dressing.

If ingested in larger amounts, apple cider vinegar can lead to low levels of potassium and osteoporosis.

People with diabetes should exercise caution when drinking this mixture. Monitor your blood sugar levels carefully throughout the day.

You shouldn't drink this mixture if you're taking:

- insulin
- digoxin (Digox)
- diuretics, such as spironolactone (Aldactone)

5. Celery juice

Celery juice is thought to clear away toxins that contribute to kidney stone formation and has long been used in traditional medications. It also helps flush out the body so you can pass the stone.

Blend one or more celery stalks with water, and drink the juice throughout the day.

You shouldn't drink this mixture if you have:

- any bleeding disorder
- low blood pressure
- a scheduled surgery

You also shouldn't drink this mixture if you're taking:

- levothyroxine (Synthroid)
- lithium (Lithane)
- medications that increase sun sensitivity, such as isotretinoin (Sotret)
- sedative medications, such as alprazolam (Xanax)

6. Pomegranate juice

Pomegranate juice has been used for centuries to improve overall kidney function. It will flush stones and other toxins from your system. It's packed with antioxidants, which help keep the kidneys healthy and may have a role in preventing kidney stones from developing.

It also lowers your urine's acidity level. Lower acidity levels reduce your risk for future kidney stones.

Pomegranate juice's effect on preventing kidney stones needs to be better studied, but there does appear to be some benefit in taking pomegranate extract, lowering the risk of stones.

There's no limit to how much pomegranate juice you can drink throughout the day.

You shouldn't drink pomegranate juice if you're taking:

- medications changed by the liver
- blood pressure medications, such as chlorothiazide (Diuril)
- rosuvastatin (Crestor)

7. Kidney bean broth

The broth from cooked kidney beans is a traditional dish, often used in India, that has been used to improve overall urinary and kidney health. It also helps dissolve and flush out the stones. Simply strain the liquid from cooked beans and drink a few glasses throughout the day.

8. Dandelion root juice

Dandelion root is a kidney tonic that stimulates the production of bile. This is thought to help eliminate waste, increase urine output, and improve digestion. Dandelions have vitamins (A, B, C, D) and minerals such as potassium, iron, and zinc.

One study showed that dandelion is effective in preventing the formation of kidney stones.

You can make fresh dandelion juice or buy it as a tea. If you make it fresh, you may also add orange peel, ginger, and apple to taste. Drink 3 to 4 cups throughout the day.

Some people experience heartburn when they eat dandelion or its parts.

You shouldn't drink this mixture if you're taking:

- blood thinners
- antacids
- antibiotics
- lithium
- diuretics, such as spironolactone (Aldactone)

Talk to your doctor before taking dandelion root extract, as it can interact with many medications.

9. Wheatgrass juice

Wheatgrass is packed with many nutrients and has long been used to enhance health. Wheatgrass increases urine flow to help pass the stones. It also contains vital nutrients that help cleanse the kidneys.

You can drink 2 to 8 ounces of wheatgrass juice per day. To prevent side effects, start with the smallest amount possible and gradually work your way up to 8 ounces.

If fresh wheatgrass juice isn't available, you can take powdered wheatgrass supplements as directed.

Taking wheatgrass on an empty stomach can reduce your risk for nausea. In some cases, it may cause appetite loss and constipation.

10. Horsetail juice

Horsetail has been used to increase urine flow to help to flush out kidney stones and can soothe swelling and inflammation. It also has antibacterial and antioxidant properties that aid in overall urinary health.

However, you shouldn't use horsetail for more than 6 weeks at a time. There are dangers of seizures, decreased levels of B vitamins, and loss of potassium.

You shouldn't use horsetail if you take lithium, diuretics, or heart medications such as digoxin.

Horsetail isn't recommended for children and pregnant or breastfeeding women. Horsetail contains nicotine and shouldn't be taken if you're using a nicotine patch or trying to quit smoking.

You also shouldn't drink horsetail juice if you have:

- alcohol use disorder
- diabetes
- low potassium levels
- low thiamine levels

WHEN TO SEE YOUR DOCTOR

See your doctor if you're unable to pass your stone within 6 weeks or you begin experiencing severe symptoms that include:

- severe pain
- blood in your urine
- fever
- chills
- nausea
- vomiting

Your doctor will determine whether you need medication or any other therapy to help you pass the stone.

FOODS TO EAT AND AVOID WHEN YOU HAVE KIDNEY STONES

Eating less animal protein can help fight the most common types of kidney stones, but it is very important for those with uric acid stones. Yes, it can be good to eat protein, but many people eat too much. With kidney stones – especially uric acid stones – you should strive to only eat about 6-8 ounces of meat, to include beef, chicken, pork or fish in one day. Picture your 6-8 ounce serving size to be about the size of your fist or a deck of cards.

Some animal protein sources lead the body to produce more uric acid than others. The ones to stay away from are those with high levels of purine. Purine causes the body to make too much uric acid. The foods to limit in the list below have very high purine levels – from 100 to 1,000 mg per 3-ounce serving. Strive to avoid these products – or cut back if one of your Favorites are on this list. Try drinking a glass of water before and after you eat to help flush-out the purines.

FOODS TO ENJOY

- Small amounts of animal-based proteins
- Milk, yogurt, cottage cheese
- Proteins in plant-based foods like peas, split peas, lentils

FOODS TO LIMIT

- Anchovies and sardines
- Mackerel and herring
- Haddock and cod
- Scallops, shrimp and mussels
- Fish roe
- Bacon
- Meat extracts like bouillon, broth and gravy
- Mincemeat, sweetbreads
- Organ meets like liver, kidney, brains, and heart
- Veal and venison
- Goose and partridge
- Yeast and yeast extract

SALT

Limit the total amount of sodium in your diet to less than 2,300 mg per day

FOODS TO ENJOY

- Herbs and spices instead of salt. Try garlic, ginger, cumin, lemon or herbs
- Frozen vegetables labeled "fresh frozen" with no added seasoning
- Fresh and frozen fruits and vegetables
- Whole grains, milk and yogurt

FOODS TO LIMIT

- Pre-packaged meals
- Processed foods: try low sodium crackers, soups, broth and canned goods
- Fast food
- Standard restaurant meals – you can ask for healthy adjustments

- Add-ons, like ketchup and salad dressing - these often are high in salt and sugar How do you fight kidney stones with food?

You may not know what type of stone you have. But, changing your diet and taking certain medications have been shown to be the best in stopping a stone from forming in the first place and keeping you from getting another one in the future. Here are some things to help you fight future kidney stones though food:

- Fluids. Drink enough fluids each day: 3 liters, or 10, 10-ounce glasses.
- Fruits & Veggies. Eat plenty every day: 5 servings each of ½ cup.
- Low Oxalate. Eat foods with low oxalate levels: only if you have high
  - urine oxalate.

- Less Meat. Eat more plant-based protein & limit meat: strive for 1 small portion a day.
- Calcium. Eat more calcium-rich foods: about 1,000 milligrams (mg) per day.
- Less Salt. Limit sodium in your diet: 2,300 mg – or 1 teaspoon of salt –
- per day.

It can be hard to change the way we eat. But changes to diet may bring great benefits. Not only can it help with kidney stones, but it may help you lower your blood pressure, blood sugar and cholesterol levels.

Remember, your health care provider will recommend you do what is best for you and the type of stones you have. Not every tip will work for every stone former. The recommendations are not a one size fits all. If you feel lifestyle and dietary changes aren't helping, talk to your health care provider.

Drinks

Drinking more fluid is a must for fighting kidney stones. The best thing you

can do to fight kidney stones is to drink more, especially water. Aim to drink a "10x10" – 10, 10-ounce glasses per day. If you're exercising, or it's hot out, drink even more!

Try to drink more with these ideas and recipes.

- Keep it close. Carry a water bottle with you so you can take sips throughout the day.
- Match with meals. Include at least one beverage with each meal.

Decaffeinated is best.

- Drinking jug. Keep a pitcher of water on the counter or in the fridge so it's handy at home and work.
- Flavor it up. Cut up lemon, lime, watermelon or mint leaves and add these to your glass of water for a refreshing flavor.
- Eat your drinks. Eat fluid-filledo foods like watermelon, honeydew melon, plums, lettuce and cucumber.
- Alarming results. Set alarms for yourself on your smart phone or pop-ups on your calendar at work.
- Lots of liquids. Try other liquids like milk, lemonade and iced tea
- (homemade with less sugar) or smoothies.
- Freeze it for fun. Freeze juice (grape, mango) into ice cubes to cool down hot tea or make a delightful drink.

- Stop time. Don't let those fruits go bad. Freeze fruits like bananas,

Strawberries, peaches, blueberries and apricots for quick access to make a great frozen smoothie.

- Fluid helps your body in many ways, it:
- Controls your heart rate and your blood pressure
- Keeps your body temperature steady
- Removes toxins and waste
- Carries nutrients and oxygen around your body
- Protects organs, tissues and joints
- Helps fight kidney stones!

KIDNEY STONE RECIPIES

PEACHY STRAWBERRY SLUSH

Drink Total: 10 m

INGREDIENTS

- 4 medium peaches, peeled, pitted and
- sliced or one can of peaches
- 1 ½ cups crushed ice
- 1 tablespoon lemon juice or lime juice
- 1 ½ cups plain seltzer water, chilled
- 5-8 fresh strawberries
- Orange peel curls (optional)

DIRECTION

1. In a blender, combine peaches, strawberries, crushed ice and lemon or lime juice.

Cover and blend until smooth.

2. Spoon fruit mixture into tall, chilled glasses; top with carbonated water. If desired,

garnish drinks by threading fresh strawberry slices on wooden skewers; wrap orange

peel curls around skewers. Place skewers in drinks. Fancy!

WATERMELON-ROSEMARY FLAVORED WATER

- Total: 8 h
- Prep: 10 m

INGREDIENTS

- 1 cup watermelon
- 2 stems fresh rosemary
- 10 cups water

DIRECTION

1. Cut watermelon into cubes.

2. Add all ingredients to a pitcher and stir.

3. Refrigerate overnight before serving.

REFRESHING CUCUMBERAND LEMON WATER

- Total: 8 h
- Prep: 10 m

INGREDIENTS

- 1 cucumber
- 1 lemon
- ¼ cup basil leaves
- ¼ cup mint leaves
- 8 cups water

DIRECTION

1. Thinly slice cucumber and lemon.

2. Finely chop basil and mint leaves.

3. Add all ingredients to a pitcher.

4. Refrigerate overnight before serving, with or without ice.

Drink more water.

When it comes to managing kidney stones, drinking more water helps. Not

drinking enough water is the #1 risk factor for developing kidney stones.

QUINOA GRITS N' EGGS

- Total: 15 m
- Prep: 5 m

INGREDIENTS

- 1 cup dry quinoa
- 1 egg
- ½ tablespoon olive oil or butter
- Small bunch parsley, chopped
- Pinch of chopped scallions

- 2 tablespoons cheddar cheese, shredded

DIRECTION

1. Rinse quinoa for about 2 minutes, using your hands.

2. Fill a medium pot with 2 cups water, add quinoa and bring to a boil. When the water boils, reduce heat to low and cover. Simmer covered 15 minutes. Remove from the heat and keep covered for a few more minutes without lifting the lid. Keep it covered until the quinoa is tender but still chewy. White spiral-like thread will appear around each grain.

3. While the quinoa is minutes from being done, heat olive oil or butter in a pan and fry your egg sunny side up so the white is set but the yolk remains runny.

4. Stir chopped parsley and scallion into the hot quinoa, then plate (about ½ per

person). Top with shredded cheddar cheese. Place egg on top. Serve.

OVEN OMLETTES

Total: 30 m Prep: 10 m

INGREDIENTS

- 10 ounces broccoli, chopped (or any other veggie)
- 4 eggs
- ¾ cup ricotta cheese
- ½ cup bell peppers, diced
- 1 scallion or green onion, chopped
- 2 drops hot sauce
- ½ teaspoon black pepper
- 8 foil baking cups

DIRECTION

Preheat oven to 350 degrees.

1. Line muffin tin with foil baking cups and spray with cooking spray

2. Whisk all ingredients in a bowl.

3. Spoon the mixture to fill each baking cup.

4. Bake 20 minutes, or until they feel firm to the touch in the center.

5. Cool 5 minutes on wire rack before eating.

6. Once cold, wrap extras in plastic wrap to store in a freezer-safe bag. You can reheat them to enjoy later.

FRESH BLUEBERRY LEMON SMOOTHIE

Total: 10 m Prep: 5 m

This high nutrient, refreshing smoothie is an easy go-to option to fill you up as you start your day. The trick is to keep frozen fresh fruits on hand.

You can slice and freeze bananas, as they get soft, or any fruit that gets too ripe. (Remove the peels before freezing.) You can also buy frozen fruit.

INGREDIENTS:

- 1 frozen banana
- ½ cup frozen blueberries
- ½ lemon, squeezed
- ½ cup frozen strawberries or mango
- ½ cup plain yogurt or milk
- For extra nutrients, add ground flax seed

DIRECTION

1. Blend all of the ingredients in a blender. Add 2 or 3 ice cubes and blend at high

speed until smooth.

2. Pour into 3 large glasses and enjoy!

PEACH AND YOGURT PARFAIT

- Total: 5 m

INGREDIENTS:

- 1 cup fat free plain yogurt
- 1 cup peach, chopped
- 3 tablespoons granola
- A few dashes of cinnamon

DIRECTION

1. Evenly layer ingredients in a tall glass.

2. Enjoy now or place in the refrigerator for up to 1 day.

WARM APPLE PIE OATMEAL

Total: 5 m

INGREDIENTS

- 1/3 cup milk

- ½ cup rolled oats
- ½ small apple, diced
- 1 dash ground cinnamon
- 1 dash ground nutmeg
- 1 teaspoon brown sugar
- Optional: 2 tablespoons shredded
- coconut or granola to garnish

DIRECTION

1. Combine milk, oats, diced apple, cinnamon and nutmeg in a large bowl. Microwave on high for 1 ½ minutes. Stir.

2. Add a small amount of brown sugar just before eating. This offers the best flavor

and helps you avoid using too much. For a little crunch, add shredded coconut or granola just before eating. Enjoy!

NO-COOK OVERNIGHT OATMEAL

Total: 8 h Prep: 5 m

INGREDIENTS

- 1/3 cup milk
- ¼ cup rolled oats
- ¼ cup Greek yogurt
- 1 teaspoon chia seeds
- 1 teaspoon honey or maple syrup
- 1 teaspoon vanilla
- 1 teaspoon ground cinnamon
- ¼ cup fresh fruit (bananas, peaches, mango, strawberries or blueberries)
- Optional: shredded coconut

DIRECTION

1. Combine milk, oats, Greek yogurt, chia seeds, honey, vanilla and cinnamon in a

half-pint jar with a lid; cover and shake until combined. Remove lid and fold in fruit.

Cover jar with lid.

2. Refrigerate overnight. Enjoy in the morning.

THREE CHEESEVEGGIE LASAGNA

Total: 1 h Prep: 15 m

INGREDIENTS

- 2 teaspoons olive oil
- 1 onion, diced
- 1 yellow squash, cubed
- 3 cloves garlic, crushed
- 5 ounce bag of kale-broccoli slaw
- (or shredded kale)
- 1 15-ounce container fat free ricotta cheese
- ½ cup low fat shredded Swiss cheese
- 3 tablespoons parmesan cheese
- 3 cups fat free milk
- 3 tablespoons all-purpose flour

- 1 package no-boil lasagna; divided into thirds
- Ground green pepper to taste as garnish

DIRECTION

Preheat the oven to 375 degrees.

1. Spray 9x13-inch baking dish with nonstickspray (olive oil spray is great).

2. Heat oil in large non-stick skillet over medium-high heat. Add onion and squash; cook, stirring occasionally, until lightly browned, about 8 minutes. Stir in kale and garlic; cook, stirring constantly, until wilted, about 3 minutes. Remove from heat; let cool 5 minutes. Stir in ricotta, Swiss & parmesan cheeses until well mixed. Set aside.

3. To make sauce, whisk together milk and flour in medium saucepan until smooth.

Cook over medium heat whisking constantly, until sauce comes to a boil and thickens, about 8 minutes.

4. Layer ingredients into baking dish: ½-cup sauce in bottom of dish, top with 1/3 of noodles (3-4 noodles), overlapping slightly and then top with ½ of veggie mixture over noodles. Repeat. The top layer will include last 1/3 of noodles and the remaining sauce.

5. Cover lasagna loosely with foil. Bake 45 minutes. Remove foil, bake until hot and bubbly, about 10 minutes. Let stand 10 minutes before serving.

KIDNEY STONE SAFE ENERGY BALLS

- PREP TIME: 10 min

INGREDIENTS

- 1.5 cup of Old fashioned oats
- 2 tbsp Lilly's stevia baking semi sweet chocolate chips
- 1 tbsp honey
- 1 cup of peanut butter

INSTRUCTIONS

1. In a large bowl mix all the ingredients together.

2. Roll into bite-size balls.

3. Put in pan and place in fridge to set.

4. They keep nicely in freezer and I like to put them there as I think about them less and therefore eat less!

NOTES

Oxalate: 14mg/Energy Ball Added Sugar: 1g
Calcium: 9mg

FRIED GNOCCHI WITHBROCCOLI AND PEAS

Total: 30 m Prep: 10 m

INGREDIENTS

- 1 pound prepared gnocchi
- 4 tablespoons extra-virgin olive oil
- 1 medium-small yellow onion, thinly
- sliced (about 1 cup)
- 2 cups chopped broccoli (frozen or fresh)
- ½ cup frozen peas
- 2 cloves diced garlic
- ¼-½ cup water
- ¼-½ teaspoons red pepper flakes
- (more or less, to taste)
- 1 teaspoons lemon zest, plus 2
- tablespoons lemon juice
- 2 tablespoons grated parmigianoreggiano; more for serving

DIRECTION

1. Bring a large saucepan of water to a boil. Add the gnocchi and cook them until they float. Drain.

2. Meanwhile, in a large (preferably 12-inch) nonstick skillet, heat 2 tablespoons oil to cook the onion over medium heat until it begins to brown. Add in the broccoli and garlic. Stir and sauté, then cover the mixture for 5 minutes or so, until the broccoli softens. Add the frozen peas and pepper flakes and sauté for another 2-3 minutes until the peas warm. Stir in the lemon zest and lemon juice. Put this mixture aside.

3. Add the remaining 2 tablespoons of oil to the skillet and add in the gnocchi. Fry the gnocchi over medium-high heat for about 5 -10 minutes, stir. Brown the gnocchi on all sides.

4. Gently mix in the onion, broccoli and pea mixture, as well as the parmigiano, along with ¼

to ½ cup water to moisten and coat the gnocchi (about 4 tablespoons).

5. Serve immediately, sprinkled with extra Parmigiano.

COMFORTING CHICKEN NOODLE SOUP

Total: 65 m Prep: 15 m

Chicken noodle soup is one of those meals that we all know and love. This one is made

with hearty chicken in a seasoned broth with wholesome vegetables and noodles.

Here's a quick and easy recipe that provides a comforting and satisfying meal.

INGREDIENTS

- 2 tablespoons unsalted butter or margarine
- ½ yellow onion chopped

- 2 carrots, sliced
- 2 stalks celery, thinly sliced
- ½ teaspoon coarse ground black pepper
- 4 cups low-sodium chicken broth
- 2 boneless, skinless chicken breasts
- 1 teaspoon fresh dill
- 8 ounces egg noodles, cooked 1 minute less than the directions

DIRECTION

1. Start by sautéing the onion in a large pot or Dutch oven. Cook over medium heat with the butter or margarine. When the onion wilts, add the celery, carrots and pepper, and sauté for another for 3-4 minutes.

2. Add broth and chicken. Bring the soup to a boil, then reduce the heat, add dill and simmer for 20 minutes. Remove the chicken and shred it into bite-size pieces.

3. Before serving, add the noodles. This lower-salt version will taste sweeter than traditional soup.

BLACK-EYED PEA SOUP

Total: 15 m* Prep: 10 m

This soup is easy to make for a nice weeknight meal. Black-eyed peas are a low-oxalate bean, so they're great to use. This tasty meal is made with 'good for you' ingredients and will help you fight kidney stones. Make it with or without chicken, based on your meat limit for the day.

INGREDIENTS

- 2 teaspoon olive oil or butter
- 2 leeks, white and light green parts only, cut into ¼-inch rounds
- ½ teaspoon dried sage

- 3 14-ounce cans reduced salt chicken broth
- 1 15-ounce can black-eyed peas, rinsed
- Optional: 3 boneless chicken breasts,
- baked and shredded

DIRECTION

1. Heat oil or butter in large pot over medium high heat.

2. Add leeks and cook, stirring until soft (about 3 minutes).

3. Stir in sage and keep cooking until aromatic (about 30 seconds).

4. Stir in broth, raise heat to high, cover and bring to a boil.

5. Add black-eyed peas (and optional chicken) and cook until heated through (about 3 minutes). Serve hot.

* Total time is based on using pre-cooked chicken.

HERBED SALMON WITH BOK CHOY

Total: 30 m Prep: 20 m

INGREDIENTS

- 4 slices of salmon (about the size of a deck of cards) rinsed with water
- 1 tablespoon olive oil
- 1 tablespoon salt-free seasoning blend
- 2 tablespoons fresh rosemary
- 4 lemon slices
- 4 tablespoons lemon juice
- ½ cup white wine

DIRECTION

Preheat the oven to 400 degrees.

1. Brush top and bottom of salmon fillets with olive oil and flavor with seasoning blend and chopped rosemary.

2. Place each piece of seasoned salmon on apiece of aluminum foil.

3. Top each piece with 1 lemon slice, 1 tablespoon of lemon juice, ½ tablespoon of wine.

4. Wrap salmon tightly in the foil packets.

5. Place the foil packets in the oven and bake for 15-20 minutes. Alternate: place foil packets on hot grill and cook for 10 minutes, flipping once.

6. Test fish to see that the fish is flaky before serving.

ENJOY THIS MAIN MEAL WITH A SIDE OF BOK CHOY

INGREDIENT

- 2 tablespoons olive oil
- 4 cups bok choy (2 bunches), rinsed well
- (especially between stalks)
- 2 cloves of garlic, chopped
- ½ cup low-salt chicken or vegetable stock
- ½ fresh lemon

DIRECTION

In a large pan, heat olive oil. Drop in the bok choy, garlic, and low-salt stock. Stir and cover to cook for 3-5 minutes until the leaves are soft, but still have a crunch. Mix occasionally. Squeeze fresh lemon on top and mix it in.

ROBUST CHICKEN CURRY

Total: 30 m Prep: 20 m

This quick and easy chicken curry is creamy, full of flavor and takes less than half an

hour to cook! The basmati rice makes the complete dish more delicious and filling.

INGREDIENTS

- ½ onion, sliced
- 1 can chickpeas, drained and rinsed
- (try a low-sodium variety)
- 1 cup cauliflower, small pieces
- 6 spring onions, chopped
- 3 cloves of garlic, diced
- 2 tablespoons vegetable oil
- Half of 1 can of low-sodium diced tomatoes
- 2 tablespoons curry powder
- 1 teaspoon ground ginger

- 4 pieces of boneless skinless chicken
- thigh, cut into 1 inch pieces
- ¼ cup water
- ¼ cup plain Greek yogurt, plus extra to serve
- Pinch of pepper
- 1 cup basmati rice

DIRECTION

1. Thinly slice the onions. Dice the garlic and cauliflower.

2. Heat oil in a large saucepan over a medium heat. Cook the onions for a few minutes. Add garlic, curry powder, ginger and chicken. Cook for 2-3 minutes on each side to coat and brown the chicken. Add a splash of water if the pan gets dry (you don't want the spices to burn).

3. Add tomatoes and ¼ cup water; boil. Reduce heat to medium-low and cook for 10-15 minutes.

It's ready when the chicken is cooked through with no sign of pink in the middle of the pieces.

4. For Rice: While the chicken cooks, prepare the rice. Pour the rice into a saucepan and rinse it under cold tap water to clean the water. Drain the cloudy water away and rinse again. Boil the rice in fresh water then cover and reduce the heat to a low simmer for 10 minutes. Remove heat and let it sit. Keep the lid on to let the rice finish cooking.

5. Take the curry off the heat. Stir in the yogurt, then season with pepper. Serve the curry with the rice and garnish with a drizzle of yogurt.

SLOW COOKER CREAM CHEESE CHICKEN CHILI

Total: 6 h Prep: 10 m

INGREDIENTS

- 2 cups dried kidney beans, soaked for
- 24 hours (or 1, 15 ounce can, rinsed)
- 1 ½ cup frozen corn
- 1 onion, diced
- 1 can diced tomatoes with green chilies
- 2 chicken breasts
- 3 tablespoons ranch seasoning
- 1 teaspoon cumin
- 1 tablespoons dark red chili powder
- 1 teaspoon onion powder
- 1 teaspoon garlic powder
- 1 cup water
- 1 8-ounce package of cream cheese

DIRECTION

1. Place frozen chicken breast in the bottom of the slow cooker. Add onion, corn, beans, canned tomatoes, water and all seasonings. Top with cream cheese.

2. Cook on low for 8 hours.

3. Shred chicken. Stir entire contents to blend and serve.

COLD TURKEY RICE SALAD

Total: 30 m* Prep: 10 m

INGREDIENTS

- 2 tablespoons rice vinegar
- 2 tablespoons lime juice
- 1 tablespoon olive oil
- 1 tablespoon honey
- 1 teaspoon ground ginger

- 3 ½ cups cooked wild or brown rice
- 1 ½ cups chopped, boneless, skinless, cooked turkey breast
- 1/3 cup dried cranberries
- 1 bunch chopped green onions (½ cup)

DIRECTION

1. Use leftover turkey from a prior meal. Or, cook turkey in advance by roasting 2 turkey cutlets in the oven. Brush with oil and place them in shallow roasting pan. Cook in oven preheated to 350 degrees for 15-20 minutes, to an internal temperature of 180 degrees. Chill and cut into small squares.

2. Cook wild or brown rice as directed in advance. Chill.

3. In a small bowl, whisk together the vinegar, lime juice, oil, honey and ginger.

4. In a large bowl, combine the rice, turkey, cranberries and green onion.

5. Toss with the ginger dressing. Refrigerate until ready to serve.

*Total time is based on using pre-cooked turkey

SLOW COOKER THAI CHICKEN

Total: 6 h Prep: 10 m

INGREDIENTS

- 13 ½ ounces unsweetened coconut milk
- 7 teaspoons Thai red curry paste
- 1 teaspoon chopped garlic
- ½ teaspoon ground ginger
- 1 head uncooked cauliflower, cut into florets
- 1 sweet red pepper, coarsely chopped
- 2 medium carrots, cut into ½ inch slices

- 1 pound chicken breast, uncooked and cut into 2-inch cubes
- 2 tablespoons sunflower seed butter (no salt variety)
- 1/3 cup fresh cilantro, chopped
- 3 medium green onions, sliced
- 1 fresh lime, cut into 6 wedges

DIRECTION

1. Cube chicken and coat with 2 teaspoons of curry paste to marinade while preparing the rest of the ingredients.

2. In a 4 to 6 quart slow cooker, add coconut milk, 2-4 more teaspoons curry paste, garlic, ginger and salt. Add cauliflower, red pepper and carrots. Mix to coat. Place chicken on top of the vegetable mixture.

3. Cover and cook on LOW setting until cooked through and veggies are tender about 5-6 hours.

4. Gently stir in sunflower seed butter and more curry paste (if you like the spice) into slow cooker until blended.

5. Stir in cilantro and green onions.

6. Spoon into bowls and serve with a lime wedge.

ORZO WITH ROASTED VEGETABLES AND FETA

Total: 40 m Prep: 15 m

INGREDIENTS

- 1 small eggplant (or squash), 1-inch diced
- 1 red bell pepper, 1-inch diced
- 1 yellow bell pepper, 1-inch diced
- 1 red onion, peeled and 1-inch diced
- 2 garlic cloves, minced
- 1 teaspoon salt-free seasoning blend
- 2 teaspoon olive oil
- ½ pound orzo or rice-shaped pasta

For the dressing:

- 1/3 cup freshly squeezed lemon juice (1-2 lemons)
- 1/3 cup olive oil
- ½ teaspoon freshly ground black pepper

For the topping:

- 4 scallions, minced (white and green parts)
- ¼ cup pignolis (pine nuts), toasted
- ¾ cup feta, crumbled (choose a lower-salt option)

DIRECTION

Preheat the oven to 425 degrees.

1. Toss the eggplant (or squash), bell peppers, onion and garlic with the olive oil, on a large sheet pan. Roast for 30 minutes, until browned, turning once with a spatula.

2. Meanwhile, cook the orzo in boiling water for 7 to 9 minutes, until tender. Drain and transfer to a large serving bowl.

3. Add the roasted vegetables to the pasta, scraping all the liquid and seasonings from the roasting pan into the pasta bowl.

4. Mix dressing together and toss into the pasta and vegetable mixture.

5. Serve, topped with scallions, pine nuts and feta.

****SIDES******

CAULIFLOWER STEAKS

Total: 30 m Prep: 10 m

INGREDIENTS

- 1 large head cauliflower, sliced lengthwise through the core into 4 'steaks'

- ¼ cup olive oil
- 1 tablespoon fresh lemon juice
- 2 cloves garlic, minced
- ½ teaspoon red pepper flakes, or to taste
- Pinch ground black or green pepper

DIRECTION

Preheat oven to 400 degrees.

1. Line a baking sheet with parchment paper.

2. Place cauliflower steaks on the prepared baking sheet.

3. Whisk olive oil, lemon juice, garlic, red pepper flakes and black pepper together in a bowl. Brush ½ of the olive oil mixture over the tops of the cauliflower steaks.

4. Roast the cauliflower steaks in the preheated oven for 15 minutes. Gently turn over each steak and brush with remaining olive oil mixture.

Continue roasting until tender and golden, 15 to 20 minutes more.

ASPARAGUS WITH LEMON SAUCE

Total: 10 m Prep: 5 m

Asparagus is a delicious, healthy springtime vegetable. It holds nutrients to help fight cancer, feed your brain and help you slim down. It is high in potassium, which is good for blood pressure and it has asparaptine, which helps improve blood flow. Try this recipe for asparagus with a creamy lemon sauce. It's a great side dish and an easy choice for people who want to fight kidney stones.

INGREDIENTS

- 20 medium asparagus spears, rinsed and trimmed
- 1 fresh lemon, rinsed (for peel and juice)

- 2 tablespoons reduced-fat mayonnaise
- 1/8 teaspoon ground black pepper

DIRECTION

1. Place 1 inch of water in a 4-quart pot with a lid. Place a steamer basket inside the pot and add asparagus. Cover and bring to a boil over highheat. Reduce heat to medium. Cook for 5-10 minutes, until asparagus is bright green and easily pierced with a sharp knife. Do not overcook.

2. While the asparagus cooks, grate the lemon zest into a small bowl. Cut the lemon in half and squeeze the juice into the bowl. Use the back of a spoon to press out extra juice and remove pits. Add mayonnaise and pepper. Stir well. Set aside.

3. When the asparagus is tender, remove the pot from the heat. Place asparagus spears in a serving bowl. Drizzle the lemon sauce evenly

over the asparagus (about 1½ teaspoons per portion) and serve.

MARKET QUINOA SALAD WITH FRESH MOZZARELLA

Total: 30 m Prep: 10 m

INGREDIENTS

- 1 cup cooked quinoa (quinoa is cooked like rice: 1 cup quinoa in 2 cups water)
- ¼ cup red onion, diced
- 1 cup cherry tomatoes, halved
- 1 cup frozen sweet peas
- 1 red bell pepper, diced
- 1 yellow pepper diced
- 1 small zucchini or cucumber, diced
- 1 round fresh mozzarella (about ¾ cup)
- 1/8 cup fresh parsley, chopped

For the Dressing (to taste):

- ½ lemon, squeezed
- 1 tablespoon orange juice
- 2 tablespoons extra virgin olive oil
- 1 ½ tablespoons balsamic vinegar
- ½ teaspoon mustard (or dry mustard for even lower sodium)
- 1 teaspoon garlic, minced
- ½ teaspoon dried oregano
- 1/8 teaspoon (or 3 grinds) fresh pepper

DIRECTION

1. Rinse quinoa for about 2 minutes, using your hands.

2. Fill a medium pot with 2 cups water, add quinoa and bring to a boil. When the water boils, reduce heat to low and cover. Simmer covered 15 minutes. Remove from the heat and keep covered for a few more minutes without lifting the lid. Keep it covered until the quinoa is tender but still chewy. White spiral-like thread will

appear around each grain. Fluff with a fork and set aside in a large mixing bowl to cool.

3. Dice all of the vegetables and mix them together. (Do not add the cheese yet.)

4. Combine the vegetables, quinoa, and add ½ of the dressing. Add the cheese and taste. Add more dressing, until you get the flavor you like.

CUCUMBER-CARROT SALAD

Total: 40 m Prep: 10 m

Try this light Asian salad when you're looking for something different. You can use a fun "spiralizer" to thinly slice the vegetables, or use pre-packaged thinly sliced carrots. More simply, you can use a handy peeler to create paper-thin vegetable slices. The vinaigrette is light and refreshing.

INGREDIENTS

- ¼ cup unseasoned rice vinegar
- 1 teaspoon sugar
- ½ teaspoon olive oil
- 1/8 teaspoon black pepper
- ½ cucumber
- 1 cup carrots
- 2 tablespoons green onion
- 2 tablespoons red bell pepper
- ½ teaspoon no-salt Italian seasoning

DIRECTION

1. Combine rice vinegar, sugar, olive oil and black pepper in a medium bowl. Stir with a whisk.

2. Cut the cucumber in half vertically, remove seeds and use a peeler, spiralizer or knife to thinly slice into thin pieces. Slice carrots and green onion. Finely chop the bell pepper.

3. Add carrots, onion, red bell pepper, cucumber and Italian seasoning to vinegar mixture; toss to coat.

4. Cover and chill 30 minutes.

CORNBREAD-BROCCOLI STUFFING

Total: 1 h 20 m Prep: 20 m

This cornbread stuffing is savory and nutritious. Broccoli adds vitamins K and C, with folate (folic acid), potassium, and fiber. Serve it with meat, fish or a vegetable-based main dish.

INGREDIENTS

Cornbread

- ¾ cup cornmeal
- 3 tablespoons all-purpose flour
- ¾ teaspoon baking powder
- ¼ teaspoon baking soda

- 1/8 teaspoon salt
- ½ cup 2 percent milk
- 1/8 teaspoon drops vinegar
- 1 egg
- 1 tablespoon canola oil Stuffing
- 1 ½ tablespoons margarine
- ¾ cup frozen broccoli (partially thaw and chop in ½" pieces)
- 2 slices white bread crust removed, torn in pieces
- 1 2/3 cups chicken broth (low sodium variety)
- ¾ teaspoon poultry seasoning
- ¼ teaspoon ground sage
- ½ teaspoon onion powder
- 1/8 teaspoon white pepper

Preheat the oven to 425 degrees.

DIRECTION

1. Combine the cornmeal, flour, baking powder, baking soda and salt in a bowl.

2. Make a well in the center.

3. In a large measuring cup, whisk together the milk, vinegar, egg and oil.

4. Pour the liquid ingredients into the well and gently stir until all is moistened.

5. Spray a 7-inch square baking dish with cooking spray.

6. Pour in the cornmeal batter and spread evenly.

7. Bake for 20 minutes or just until golden and the center springs back when touched.

To make the stuffing:

1. In a large mixing bowl, combine the cornbread (crumbled) and white bread pieces.

2. In a saucepan, over medium heat, sauté the broccoli and butter until tender – do not brown.

3. Combine the sautéed broccoli with the bread mixture. Stir in chicken broth, using enough to moisten. Stir in the seasonings and blend well.

4. Spread the mixture in a large shallow baking dish measuring about 10" x 15".

5. Bake for 20-30 minutes.

ROASTED SPRING VEGETABLES

Total: 30 m Prep: 10 m

You can add fresh, colorful and richly flavored vegetables to any meal with this super easy recipe. It is full of nutrients, low in sodium and oxalates and has no added sugar or no uric acid. Roasting vegetables "wakes-up" their flavors.

Add these roasted vegetables to a bed of lettuce and you can enjoy a light, but filling lunch.

INGREDIENTS

- 6 carrots, quartered lengthwise
- 1 bunch of asparagus, ends trimmed
- 1 head of broccoli, cut or broken into medium pieces
- 1 head of cauliflower, cut or broken into medium pieces
- 2 leeks, green ends removed, halved lengthwise, and divided into three chunks
- 2 tablespoons olive oil
- ½ teaspoon ground black pepper
- ¼ teaspoon paprika
- ¼ teaspoon garlic powder
- 1 tablespoon fresh lemon juice
- Pinch of salt-free seasoning mix

DIRECTION

Preheat the oven to 425 degrees.

1. On a baking pan lined with parchment paper, place the carrots and sprinkle 1 tablespoon of olive oil on them. Mix the carrots in the oil so everything is coated. Roast for 10 minutes.

2. While the carrots cook, mix the asparagus, broccoli, cauliflower and leeks in the remaining olive oil.

3. Take out the carrots and spread the remaining vegetables into the pan. Season the tops of the vegetables with pepper, paprika, garlic powder and lemon juice. Return to the oven and roast for another 20-25 minutes. Stir the mixture ½ way through.

4. Remove from the oven sprinkle with a pinch of no-salt seasoning, mix well and serve.

HOMEMADE RANCH DIP

Total: 5-10

Typically, store bought dips are full of hidden sodium. In this easy recipe, there's only 4 mg of sodium and added calcium. You can serve it as a dip or a salad dressing.

INGREDIENTS AND DIRECTIONS

(Simply mix everything together):

- 1 cup Greek Yogurt (pick a
- low-sodium variety)
- ½ teaspoon dried or fresh dill
- ½ teaspoon dried parsley
- ¼ teaspoon garlic powder
- ½ teaspoon dried minced onions
- Pinch of black pepper

CRUSTLESS ZUCCHINI QUICHE

You'll fall in love with this easy, flavorful quiche. Zucchini, onions and green chiles fill this quiche with flavor. Cottage cheese and mozzarella cheese add a delicious creaminess and great way to get in dairy!

- Prep Time15 mins
- Cook Time40 mins

INGREDIENTS

- 1 zucchini grated
- 1 small onion chopped
- 4 eggs
- 2 cups part-skim mozzarella cheese shredded
- 1 cup low-fat, reduced sodium cottage cheese
- 1 4.5oz can green chiles
- 1/2 teaspoon black pepper
- 1/4 cup green onion chopped

INSTRUCTIONS

1. Preheat oven to 375'F. Spray a 9-inch pie plate with cooking spray.

2. Press grated zucchini into paper towels to absorb as much liquid as possible.

3. Heat a medium skillet over medium-high heat and spray with cooking spray. Add onion and cook until softened, about 5 minutes. Add zucchini and cook until softened, about 3 minutes. Set aside.

4. In a large bowl, whisk eggs until thick and fluffy. Add mozzarella, cottage cheese, chiles, pepper and cooked zucchini mixture. Stir to combine.

5. Pour into prepared pie plate. Bake 35-40 minutes until top is puffed and golden brown and a toothpick inserted into the center of the quiche comes out clean.

6. Garnish with green onion.

BLUEBERRY BAKED OATMEAL

Warm, cozy, and oh so filling! We love to start our day off with this simple baked oatmeal.

- PREP5 minutes
- COOK30 minutes

INGREDIENTS

- 1 ½ cups rolled oats
- ½ cup milk
- 1/3 cup brown sugar
- ¼ cup melted butter
- 2 large eggs, beaten
- 1 teaspoon baking powder
- 1 teaspoon cinnamon
- 1 teaspoon vanilla extract
- ¾ teaspoon salt
- 1 cup blueberries, fresh or frozen

INSTRUCTIONS

1. Preheat oven to 350 degrees. Spray an 8x8 baking dish with non-stick spray.

2. Add all of the ingredients except for the blueberries to a mixing bowl and stir well to combine.

3. Fold in the blueberries gently so as not to break them up too much.

4. Spread mixture into the prepared baking dish and bake for 30 minutes or until a knife comes out mostly clean with just a few moist crumbs.

5. Spoon into bowls and serve with additional blueberries and a drizzle of cream or syrup, if desired.

EGG ROLL IN A BOWL

This quick and easy recipe will satisfy your take-out craving without the salt! Tasty cabbage, chicken and mushrooms flavored with ginger, garlic and soy sauce topped with crispy wonton strips.

- Prep Time10 mins
- Cook Time20 mins

INGREDIENTS

- 2 tsp sesame oil divided
- 1 lb ground chicken
- 14 oz bag coleslaw mix
- 8 oz white mushrooms sliced
- 4 cloves garlic chopped & divided
- 4 green onions sliced, whites & green separated
- 2 tbsp white vinegar
- 2 tbsp low sodium soy sauce
- 1 tbsp fresh ginger grated

- 1 lime
- 1 tsp Sriracha (or your favorite hot sauce)
- 1 tsp cornstarch
- 3/4 cup fried wonton strips

INSTRUCTIONS

1. In a large sided skillet, heat 1 teaspoon of sesame oil over medium high heat. Add chicken and cook until browned.

2. Add coleslaw mix, mushrooms, garlic and white parts of green onion. Cook until cabbage is tender, about 10 minutes.

3. Meanwhile, prepare sauce. Whisk vinegar, soy sauce, ginger, juice from 1/2 the lime, Sriracha and cornstarch together.

4. Add sauce to chicken & cabbage mixture. Cook 1-2 minutes, until well combined.

5. Serve garnished with sliced green parts of green onion, lime wedges and 2 tablespoons

wonton strips per serving. Serve over rice if desired. Enjoy!

CRISPY FALAFEL

- Prep Time: 20 minutes
- Cook Time: 30 minutes

This homemade falafel recipe is absolutely delicious, and remarkably crispy! Be sure to allow 4 hours soaking time for the chickpeas, preferably overnight. Then, the falafel mixture is super easy to make in a food processor. Recipe yields 12 to 13 falafels (see notes on how to double).

INGREDIENTS

- ¼ cup + 1 tablespoon extra-virgin olive oil
- 1 cup dried (uncooked/raw) chickpeas, rinsed, picked over and soaked for at least

4 hours and up to 24 hours in the
refrigerator

- ½ cup roughly chopped red onion (about
  ½ small red onion)
- ½ cup packed fresh parsley (mostly leaves
  but small stems are ok)
- ½ cup packed fresh cilantro (mostly leaves
  but small stems are ok)
- 4 cloves garlic, quartered
- 1 teaspoon fine sea salt
- ½ teaspoon (about 25 twists) freshly
  ground black pepper
- ½ teaspoon ground cumin
- ¼ teaspoon ground cinnamon

INSTRUCTIONS

1. With an oven rack in the middle position,
preheat oven to 375 degrees Fahrenheit. Pour ¼
cup of the olive oil into a large, rimmed baking
sheet and turn until the pan is evenly coated.

2. In a food processor, combine the soaked and drained chickpeas, onion, parsley, cilantro, garlic, salt, pepper, cumin, cinnamon, and the remaining 1 tablespoon of olive oil. Process until smooth, about 1 minute.

3. Using your hands, scoop out about 2 tablespoons of the mixture at a time. Shape the falafel into small patties, about 2 inches wide and ½ inch thick. Place each falafel on your oiled pan.

4. Bake for 25 to 30 minutes, carefully flipping the falafels halfway through baking, until the falafels are deeply golden on both sides. These falafels keep well in the refrigerator for up to 4 days, or in the freezer for several months.

RED ONION AND BUTTON MUSHROOM OMELETTE

MUSHROOM OMELETTE

- **INGREDIENTS**

- 4 Eggs
- 2 cloves of garlic, minced
- ½ of green bell pepper, finely chopped
- 1/2 red onion, finely chopped
- 8 button mushrooms, sliced
- Salt and pepper to taste

METHOD

Put some vegetable oil in a pan and heat it. Add your red onion, green bell pepper and garlic and allow this to sauté until soft and fragrant. Add your sliced button mushrooms and let this cook down for about 3-5 minutes until they slightly soften and shrink. Take from heat and set aside.

These are the same mushrooms I had left over after making this other BOMB mushroom dish and I bought them from Nakumatt. I am totally addicted to mushrooms!!

Whisk your eggs with the salt and pepper and add to the heated pan. This should be followed immediately by the mushroom sautee. Do not allow the eggs to set before adding the mushroom. The egg should set while the mushroom is already on it so that it does not slide off.

HONEY MUSTARD SALMON

- Prep Time5 mins
- Cook Time18 mins

INGREDIENTS

- 3 Tbs white vinegar
- 1 Tbs sugar

- 3 Tbs Dijon mustard
- 1 1/2 tsp dry mustard
- 3 Tbs canola oil
- 4 4oz salmon fillets
- 1 tsp dried thyme
- 1/2 tsp black pepper
- 1/2 cup breadcrumbs

INSTRUCTIONS

1. Whisk together vinegar, sugar, Dijon mustard and dry mustard. Slowly whisk in oil.

2. Preheat oven to 375°F.

3. Season salmon with thyme and black pepper. Spread 1 Tbs mustard sauce over each piece of salmon. Press breadcrumbs onto fish.

4. Place salmon on baking sheet. Bake salmon until crispy and golden brown,approximately 18 minutes.

5. Serve remaining mustard sauce on the side.

LOW SODIUM STIR FRY

Flavorful low sodium pork stir fry with lots of yummy veggies!

- Prep Time45 mins
- Cook Time20 mins

INGREDIENTS

- 3/4 pound pork tenderloin thinly sliced
- 1/2 head broccoli cut into florets
- 1 red bell pepper sliced
- 1 8 oz can water chestnuts drained
- 2 Tbs low sodium soy sauce
- 2 teaspoons vegetable oil
- 2 cloves garlic minced
- 2 inches fresh ginger peeled and grated
- 2 green onions chopped
- 1 cup low sodium chicken broth
- 2 tablespoons cornstarch
- 2 tablespoons low sodium soy sauce
- 2 tablespoons hoisin sauce

- 2 tablespoons dry sherry
- 3 cups brown rice cooked

Instructions

1. Combine first low sodium soy sauce (2 tablespoons) with vegetable oil, garlic, ginger and green onion. Add pork to marinade. Let sit 30 minutes.

2. Meanwhile, blanch broccoli. Make sauce by whisking together broth, cornstarch, additional 2 tablespoons low sodium soy sauce, hoisin sauce and sherry. Set aside.

3. Drain marinade from pork. Discard the marinade.

4. Heat 1 teaspoon of vegetable oil in a skillet. Add pork and cook until opaque, about 1 minute. Transfer to a plate.

5. Heat another teaspoon of vegetable oil in a skillet and add broccoli, peppers and water

chestnuts. Stir fry until tender crisp. Add pork and sauce. Continue to cook until sauce thickens, about 3 minutes.

6. Serve 1 cup stir fry over 1/2 cup rice. Garnish with additional green onion if desired.

GRILLED CHICKEN WITH MANGO AVOCADO SALSA

Spiced grilled chicken breasts topped with a sweet and tangy mango avocado salsa.

- Cook Time: 10 minutes
- Total Time: 15 minutes

INGREDIENTS

- 4 thin boneless skinless chicken breasts
- 2 teaspoons olive oil
- 2 teaspoons chili powder
- salt to taste
- 1 cup diced mango

- 1 cup diced avocado
- the juice of 1 lime
- 1/2 cup minced red bell pepper
- 1/4 cup chopped cilantro

INSTRUCTIONS

1. Heat a grill over medium-high heat. Drizzle the olive oil over the chicken breasts and sprinkle with the chili powder and salt to taste.

2. Grill for 4-5 minutes on each side or until cooked through.

3. While the chicken is cooking, combine the mango, avocado, red bell pepper and cilantro in a bowl. Stir in the lime juice and salt to taste.

4. Spoon the salsa over the chicken and serve.

MEDITERRANEAN CHICKPEA SALAD BOWL

This Mediterranean Chickpea Salad is a light a fresh dish with delicious flavor. Packed with veggies, herbs and the perfect dressing to go with it. Serve up the best healthy vegetarian Mediterranean bowl today!

PREP TIME10 minutes

INGREDIENTS

Mediterranean Chickpea Salad

- 15.5 oz can chickpeas, drained
- 1 cup cucumbers, diced
- 1 cup cherry tomatoes, halved
- 3/4 cup parsley leaves, diced
- 1/3 cup red onion, diced
- 1/4 cup feta crumbles

Dressing

- 2 garlic cloves, minced

- 2 tbsp lemon, juice of
- 3 tbsp olive oil
- 2 tbsp red wine vinegar
- 1/2 tsp dried oregano
- 1/2 tsp agave (can sub sugar)
- salt to taste (I used about a 1/2 tsp)

For the Bowl

- 1/2 cup quinoa, cooked, or more as needed
- 1/2 cup arugula, or more as needed
- 1 heaping spoonful roasted garlic hummus
- 1 warm pita bread, cut in triangles

INSTRUCTIONS

1. In a large bowl toss together chickpeas, tomatoes, cucumbers, onion, parsley, and feta.

2. Make the dressing, in a small jar whisk together minced garlic, lemon juice, olive oil, red wine vinegar, oregano, agave, and salt.

3. Pour dressing over salad and toss. Enjoy

4. To make a nourish bowl serve over quinoa and arugula. Top with hummus and warm pita bread.

ROASTED GARLICKY BRUSSELS SPROUTS

Savory, mustard-garlic Brussels. You won't be able to help yourself from going back for more!

- Prep Time5 mins
- Cook Time25 mins

INGREDIENTS

- 8 oz (about 25 sprouts) Brussels sprouts trimmed & halved
- 2 Tbs white vinegar

- 2 tsp honey
- 2 tsp Dijon mustard
- 1/8 tsp black pepper
- 1 dash salt
- 1 clove garlic minced
- 2 Tbs olive oil

INSTRUCTIONS

1. Place Brussels Sprouts on baking sheet. Recommended: Crowd sprouts ontoone side of sheet to prevent drying out.

2. Roast sprouts at 400°F for 20-25 minutes or until fork-tender.

3. Meanwhile, combine remaining ingredients.

4. When sprouts are done, combine with dressing.

THAI CUCUMBER SALAD

- prep time: 10 MINUTES

This Thai Cucumber Salad is light, refreshing and full of flavor made with simple ingredients. This refreshing salad is the perfect side dish.

INGREDIENTS

- 1/3 cup rice vinegar
- 2 Tbsp sugar
- 1/2 tsp toasted sesame oil
- 1/4 tsp red pepper flakes
- 1/2 tsp salt
- 2 large cucumbers (peeled and sliced)
- 3 green onions (diced)
- 1/4 cup chopped peanuts

INSTRUCTIONS

To start, peel and slice your cucumbers long wise. Scoop out of the seeds and then slice the cucumbers. Place the cucumbers in a bowl.

In a small bowl, make your dressing. The Sesame Oil adds so much flavor, even though you just need a little bit. Mix together vinegar, sugar, oil, red pepper flakes and salt.

Pour the dressing over the cucumbers. Garnish with sliced green onions and peanuts.

Toss everything together.

Serve your Thai Cucumber Salad immediately or I personally like to let it refrigerate for a bit.

PARMESAN ROASTED BROCCOLI

- PREP TIME10 mins
- COOK TIME30 mins

INGREDIENTS

- 1 pound broccoli
- 2 tablespoons oil
- ½ teaspoon garlic powder

- ¼ teaspoon salt
- ⅛ teaspoon pepper
- ½ cup parmesan cheese (shredded)

INSTRUCTIONS

1. Preheat oven to 400 degrees and prepare a baking sheet with nonstick cooking spray.

2. Chop broccoli and place them in a mixing bowl. Toss to coat in oil then season and toss to coat again.

3. Place broccoli on your prepared baking sheet and top with shredded parmesan cheese.

4. Bake for 25-30 minutes or until broccoli is tender.

CRISPY STUFFED ZUCCHINI

- PREP:10 MINS
- COOK:25 MINS

- 4 large zucchini halved lengthwise
- 2/3 cup panko breadcrumbs
- 1/2 cup fresh grated parmesan cheese
- ¼ cup finely chopped parsley
- 4 cloves garlic , minced
- 1/4 cup melted butter
- Salt and pepper

INSTRUCTIONS

1. Preheat oven to 400°F (200°C). Spray a baking tray or sheet with non stick cooking oil spray.

2. Arrange zucchini halves, cut side up, on the baking sheet. Set aside.

3. Mix together the breadcrumbs, parmesan cheese, parsley and garlic in a small bowl.

4. Pour in the melted butter, season with ¾ teaspoon salt and ⅓ teaspoon pepper (or to taste). Mix the ingredients together until the

breadcrumbs absorb the butter (about 40 seconds).

5. Spoon the mixture over each zucchini half, to evenly cover. Spray the topping with a little cooking oil spray.

6. Bake for 20 minutes in the hot oven until the crust is golden and the zucchini halves are cooked through.

7. Broil for a further 5 minutes on medium heat to crisp the topping.

8. Garnish with parsley and serve as a side accompaniment to any main dish.

VANILLA PANNA COTTA

INGREDIENTS

- Cooking spray
- 1 1/2 cups whole milk (see Ingredient Notes)

- 3 teaspoons powdered gelatin
- 1/3 cup sugar
- 1 1/2 cups light or heavy cream
- 1 teaspoon pure vanilla extract
- Pinch salt

INSTRUCTIONS

1. Lightly grease the ramekins: Spray the ramekins with cooking spray, then use a paper towel to wipe out most of the oil, leaving only a light residue.

2. Bloom the gelatin: Pour the milk into the saucepan and sprinkle the powdered gelatin evenly over top. Let soften for 5 minutes or until the surface of the milk is wrinkled and the gelatin grains look wet and slightly dissolved.

3. Dissolve the gelatin over low heat: Set the saucepan over low heat and warm the milk gently, stirring or whisking frequently. The milk should never boil or simmer; if you see steam,

remove the pot from the stove and let it cool down. The milk should get hot, but not so hot that you can't leave your finger in the pot for a few seconds. The gelatin will dissolve quickly as the milk warms; it melts at body temperature so this step should go quickly.

4. Check to make sure the gelatin is dissolved: After about 2 minutes of warming, rub a bit of the milk between your fingers to make sure it's smooth. Or dip a spoon in the milk and check the back for distinct grains of gelatin.

5. Dissolve the sugar: Stir the sugar into the milk and continue warming until it dissolves as well. It shouldn't take more than 5 minutes total to dissolve both the gelatin and sugar. Again, never let the mixture boil.

6. Whisk in the cream and flavorings: Remove the saucepan from the heat. Whisk in the cream, vanilla, and a pich of salt.

7. Pour into the ramekins and chill: Divide the mixture evenly between the prepared ramekins and put in the refrigerator to chill. If serving straight from the cups, without unmolding, chill for 1 to 2 hours. If you want to unmold the panna cotta, chill for at least 4 hours or overnight.

8. Prepare to unmold: Fill a large bowl partway with warm to hot water. Wipe a dessert plate with a damp paper towel (a damp plate lets you reposition the panna cotta more easily if it doesn't fall in the right spot).

9. Release the panna cotta edge from the cup: Run a thin knife carefully around the sides of a ramekin. Don't slide the knife all the way into the cup; just release the top edge of the pudding from the edge of the cup. Dip the ramekin in the warm water up to its rim, and hold it there for about 3 seconds.

10. Unmold on a plate: Invert the ramekin over the plate and shake gently to help the panna cotta fall out, or press gently on one side to help nudge it out. It should fall out on the plate easily. (If it does not, return to the warm water bath in increments of 2 seconds.) Reposition on the plate if desired. Serve immediately, or refrigerate, lightly covered, for up to 5 days. The gelatin gets stronger as it sits, so this will be a bit rubbery by days 4 or 5, but you can mitigate this by letting the panna cotta sit at room temperature for about half an hour before serving.

Printed in Great Britain
by Amazon

21799386R00076